Table Of Contents

Chapter 1: Introduction to Water Fasting and Autophagy

Understanding Water Fasting and Autophagy

Water fasting and autophagy are two powerful tools that can be utilized for weight loss, detoxification, anti-aging benefits, mental clarity, muscle preservation, spiritual growth, metabolism improvement, unhealthy eating habit reset, disease prevention, and more. In this chapter, we will delve deeper into the relationship between water fasting and autophagy, and how they work hand in hand to help individuals achieve their health and wellness goals.

Water fasting is the practice of consuming only water for a set period of time, usually ranging from 24 hours to several days. During a water fast, the body is able to enter a state of autophagy, which is the natural process of cellular self-cleansing and recycling. Autophagy plays a crucial role in removing damaged and dysfunctional cells, promoting overall cell health and longevity. By combining water fasting with autophagy, individuals can effectively cleanse their bodies at a cellular level and kickstart their weight loss journey.

For people that are trying to cleanse and lose weight, understanding the relationship between water fasting and autophagy is essential. When the body is in a state of autophagy, it becomes more efficient at burning fat for energy, which can lead to accelerated weight loss results. Additionally, autophagy can help preserve muscle mass during fasting, ensuring that the body maintains its strength and functionality while shedding excess fat. By harnessing the power of autophagy through water fasting, individuals can achieve their weight loss goals in a healthy and sustainable manner.

In addition to weight loss, water fasting and autophagy have a range of other benefits that can positively impact overall health and well-being. Autophagy has been linked to anti-aging benefits, as it helps to repair and regenerate cells, reducing the signs of aging on the skin and in the body. Water fasting can also improve mental clarity and focus, as the body is able to detoxify and reset from the effects of processed foods and toxins. By incorporating water fasting and autophagy into a regular health routine, individuals can experience improved metabolism, disease prevention, and spiritual growth.

Overall, understanding the connection between water fasting and autophagy is key for individuals looking to cleanse their bodies, lose weight, and improve their overall health. By incorporating these practices into their daily routine, individuals can harness the power of autophagy to promote cellular health, accelerate weight loss, improve mental clarity, and achieve a range of other health benefits. Whether you are a beginner to water fasting or looking to take your fasting routine to the next level, the combination of water fasting and autophagy is a powerful tool for achieving your health and wellness goals.

Benefits of Water Fasting and Autophagy for Weight Loss

Water fasting and autophagy have been gaining popularity in recent years as effective methods for weight loss and overall health improvement. When combined, these two practices can provide numerous benefits for those looking to cleanse their bodies and shed excess pounds. One of the key advantages of water fasting is its ability to kickstart the process of autophagy, which is the body's natural mechanism for cleaning out damaged cells and regenerating new, healthy ones.

Autophagy is particularly beneficial for weight loss as it helps to break down stored fat and convert it into energy. This can lead to a significant reduction in body fat percentage and an increase in lean muscle mass. By promoting autophagy through water fasting, individuals can see faster and more sustainable results in their weight loss journey.

In addition to weight loss, water fasting and autophagy have been shown to have a range of other health benefits. These include improved mental clarity and focus, detoxification of the body, anti-aging effects, and disease prevention. By allowing the body to enter a state of ketosis through fasting, individuals can also experience a boost in metabolism and increased energy levels.

For beginners looking to try water fasting and autophagy for weight loss, it is important to start slowly and gradually increase the duration of fasting periods. It is also crucial to stay hydrated and listen to your body's signals throughout the process. Consulting with a healthcare professional before starting any fasting regimen is recommended, especially for individuals with underlying health conditions.

Overall, water fasting and autophagy can be powerful tools for those seeking to cleanse their bodies, lose weight, and improve their overall health. By understanding the benefits of these practices and incorporating them into a balanced lifestyle, individuals can achieve their weight loss goals and experience lasting changes in their health and well-being.

Chapter 2: Water Fasting for Beginners

How to Start a Water Fast Safely

Starting a water fast can be a daunting task, especially if you are new to the concept. However, with the right approach, you can safely embark on this journey towards cleansing and weight loss. Here are some tips on how to start a water fast safely.

First and foremost, it is important to consult with a healthcare professional before starting a water fast, especially if you have any underlying health conditions. They can provide guidance on whether a water fast is suitable for you and how to go about it safely.

When starting a water fast, it is crucial to ease into it gradually. Begin by reducing your intake of solid foods and increasing your intake of water and other liquids. This will help prepare your body for the fast and minimize any potential side effects.

During the fast, it is important to stay hydrated by drinking plenty of water throughout the day. Aim to drink at least eight glasses of water daily to help flush out toxins from your body and keep you feeling energized.

Listen to your body during the fast and pay attention to any signs of discomfort or weakness. If you experience severe symptoms such as dizziness, nausea, or fainting, it is important to break the fast and seek medical attention immediately.

In conclusion, starting a water fast safely requires careful planning and preparation. By consulting with a healthcare professional, easing into the fast gradually, staying hydrated, and listening to your body, you can embark on this journey towards cleansing and weight loss with confidence and peace of mind.

Tips for a Successful Water Fasting Experience

Water fasting can be an incredibly effective tool for cleansing the body and losing weight quickly. However, in order to have a successful water fasting experience, it is important to follow certain tips and guidelines. Here are some tips for a successful water fasting experience:

1. Preparation is key: Before starting a water fast, it is important to prepare your body for the experience. This includes gradually reducing your intake of solid foods in the days leading up to the fast, as well as staying hydrated and getting plenty of rest. By preparing your body in this way, you can help minimize any potential side effects of the fast.

2. Stay hydrated: During a water fast, it is essential to drink plenty of water to stay hydrated. Water helps to flush toxins out of the body and can also help to curb hunger pangs. Aim to drink at least 8-10 glasses of water per day, and consider adding a pinch of Himalayan salt to your water to help maintain electrolyte balance.

3. Listen to your body: While it is normal to experience some discomfort during a water fast, it is important to listen to your body and take care of yourself. If you start to feel dizzy, weak, or lightheaded, it may be a sign that you need to break your fast. Pay attention to how you are feeling and don't push yourself beyond your limits.

4. Break your fast slowly: When it comes time to break your water fast, it is important to do so slowly and carefully. Start by introducing small amounts of easily digestible foods, such as fruits, vegetables, and soups. Avoid heavy or processed foods, as these can be hard on your digestive system after a period of fasting.

5. Follow up with healthy eating habits: After completing a water fast, it is important to continue to eat a healthy, balanced diet in order to maintain the benefits of the fast. Focus on whole, nutrient-dense foods such as fruits, vegetables, lean proteins, and whole grains. By incorporating healthy eating habits into your daily routine, you can help to support your weight loss goals and overall health.

Chapter 3: Autophagy and Weight Loss

How Autophagy Affects Weight Loss

Autophagy is a natural process in the body that plays a crucial role in weight loss. When you engage in water fasting, you are essentially triggering autophagy to kick into high gear. During this process, your body starts to break down and recycle old and damaged cells, including fat cells. This can lead to significant weight loss as your body becomes more efficient at burning fat for energy.

One of the key ways that autophagy affects weight loss is by increasing your metabolism. As your body breaks down old cells and clears out toxins, your metabolism is boosted, allowing you to burn more calories throughout the day. This can help you shed excess weight more quickly and efficiently than traditional diet and exercise alone.

Additionally, autophagy can help to preserve muscle mass during weight loss. When you engage in water fasting and trigger autophagy, your body targets damaged cells and tissues for recycling, rather than breaking down healthy muscle tissue. This can help you maintain muscle mass while losing fat, leading to a more toned and lean physique.

Furthermore, autophagy can have a profound impact on your overall health and well-being. By clearing out old and damaged cells, autophagy can help to prevent diseases such as cancer, diabetes, and heart disease. It can also improve your immune function and reduce inflammation in the body, leading to better overall health and vitality.

In conclusion, understanding how autophagy affects weight loss is crucial for anyone looking to cleanse and lose weight. By engaging in water fasting and triggering autophagy, you can boost your metabolism, preserve muscle mass, and improve your overall health. This powerful process can help you achieve your weight loss goals more quickly and efficiently, while also promoting long-term health and well-being.

Maximizing Autophagy for Weight Loss Results

In the quest for weight loss and overall health, maximizing autophagy through strategies like water fasting can be a powerful tool. Autophagy is the body's natural process of cleaning out damaged cells and regenerating new, healthy ones. By promoting autophagy, you can enhance your body's ability to burn fat, improve metabolism, and boost energy levels. In this subchapter, we will explore how you can optimize autophagy to achieve your weight loss goals effectively.

One of the most effective ways to maximize autophagy for weight loss results is through water fasting. Water fasting involves abstaining from all food and drink except water for a specified period. This practice triggers autophagy by depriving the body of nutrients, forcing it to break down and recycle damaged cells for energy. By incorporating regular water fasting into your weight loss regimen, you can promote autophagy and accelerate fat loss.

For beginners, it is essential to start slowly with water fasting to allow your body to adjust gradually. Begin with short fasts of 12-24 hours and gradually increase the duration as you become more comfortable. It is also crucial to stay hydrated during water fasting to support the detoxification process and prevent dehydration. By easing into water fasting and staying hydrated, you can optimize autophagy and achieve sustainable weight loss results.

In addition to weight loss, autophagy can also have anti-aging benefits by promoting cellular regeneration and reducing oxidative stress. By maximizing autophagy through practices like water fasting, you can slow down the aging process and maintain a youthful appearance. Furthermore, autophagy plays a vital role in disease prevention by removing toxins and waste products from cells, reducing the risk of chronic illnesses. By harnessing the power of autophagy through water fasting, you can not only lose weight but also improve your overall health and well-being.

In conclusion, maximizing autophagy through water fasting is a highly effective strategy for weight loss and overall health. By promoting cellular regeneration, boosting metabolism, and enhancing energy levels, autophagy can help you achieve your weight loss goals efficiently. Whether you are looking to reset unhealthy eating habits, improve mental clarity, or prevent disease, incorporating regular water fasting into your routine can have a profound impact on your health and well-being. Embrace the power of autophagy and unlock its potential for optimal weight loss results.

Chapter 4: Water Fasting for Detoxification

Detoxifying the Body Through Water Fasting

Water fasting is a powerful tool for detoxifying the body and promoting weight loss. By abstaining from food and only consuming water for a period of time, you give your digestive system a much-needed break and allow your body to focus on cleansing and repairing itself. This process, known as autophagy, is essential for removing toxins and damaged cells from the body, leading to improved overall health and well-being.

For people that are trying to cleanse and lose weight, water fasting can be a game-changer. Not only does it help to reset unhealthy eating habits, but it also promotes fat loss and increases metabolic rate. During a water fast, the body switches to burning stored fat for energy, leading to rapid weight loss. Additionally, autophagy plays a key role in preserving muscle mass during fasting, ensuring that the body maintains its strength and functionality.

In addition to its weight loss benefits, water fasting is also known for its detoxification properties. As the body enters a state of autophagy, it begins to break down and eliminate damaged cells and toxins, allowing for a deep cleanse at the cellular level. This process not only helps to rid the body of harmful substances but also promotes overall health and vitality.

Furthermore, water fasting has been shown to have anti-aging effects, thanks to the regenerative properties of autophagy. By removing damaged cells and promoting the growth of new, healthy cells, fasting can help to slow down the aging process and improve skin health. Additionally, autophagy has been linked to disease prevention, as it helps to boost the immune system and protect against chronic illnesses.

Overall, water fasting is a powerful tool for cleansing the body, promoting weight loss, and improving overall health. By incorporating regular fasting periods into your routine, you can reap the benefits of autophagy and enjoy a renewed sense of well-being. Whether you are looking to lose weight, detoxify your body, or simply improve your health, water fasting is a safe and effective option for achieving your goals.

Cleansing the System with Water Fasting

Water fasting is an ancient practice that has been used for centuries to cleanse the body and promote overall health and well-being. In today's modern world, where processed foods and environmental toxins are rampant, water fasting has become increasingly popular as a way to detoxify the body and jumpstart weight loss. By abstaining from solid food and consuming only water for a set period of time, the body is able to enter a state of autophagy, where it begins to break down and recycle damaged cells and proteins.

Autophagy is a natural process in the body that helps to clean out damaged cells and regenerate new, healthy ones. During water fasting, the body is able to activate autophagy more efficiently, leading to numerous health benefits. Not only does autophagy help to promote weight loss by burning fat for energy, but it also has anti-aging effects, improves mental clarity and focus, and can even help to prevent disease.

For beginners looking to try water fasting for the first time, it is important to start slow and gradually increase the duration of the fast. Beginning with a 24-hour fast and working up to longer fasts of 48 hours or more can help the body adjust and prevent any negative side effects. It is also important to stay hydrated and listen to your body during the fast, breaking the fast with light, easily digestible foods to avoid digestive upset.

One of the key benefits of water fasting is its ability to reset unhealthy eating habits. By abstaining from solid food for a period of time, the body is able to break free from cravings and dependence on processed foods, making it easier to adopt a healthier diet in the long run. Water fasting can also help to improve metabolism and promote muscle preservation during fasting, making it an effective tool for weight loss and overall health.

In addition to its physical benefits, water fasting can also have profound spiritual effects, helping to promote mindfulness, clarity, and a sense of connection to the world around us. By giving the body a break from constant digestion and allowing it to heal and regenerate, water fasting can help to promote a sense of calm and inner peace. Overall, water fasting and autophagy are powerful tools for cleansing the body, promoting weight loss, and achieving optimal health and well-being.

Chapter 5: Autophagy and Anti-Aging Benefits

The Role of Autophagy in Anti-Aging

Autophagy, the natural process by which our bodies clean out damaged cells and regenerate new, healthy ones, plays a crucial role in anti-aging. As we age, our cells accumulate damaged proteins and organelles, leading to cellular dysfunction and ultimately, aging. By activating autophagy through practices like water fasting, we can help our bodies eliminate these damaged cells and promote cellular rejuvenation, effectively slowing down the aging process.

When we engage in water fasting, our bodies enter a state of autophagy where our cells begin to break down and recycle old and damaged components. This process not only helps to cleanse our bodies of toxins and waste but also stimulates the production of new, healthy cells. By promoting autophagy through water fasting, we can effectively turn back the clock on aging and improve our overall health and vitality.

Studies have shown that autophagy can help to combat age-related diseases such as Alzheimer's, Parkinson's, and cancer by removing damaged proteins and organelles that contribute to disease progression. By incorporating water fasting into our routine, we can activate autophagy and reduce our risk of developing these debilitating conditions, allowing us to live longer, healthier lives.

In addition to its anti-aging benefits, autophagy has also been shown to support weight loss by promoting fat metabolism and preserving lean muscle mass during fasting. By activating autophagy through practices like water fasting, we can enhance our body's ability to burn fat for fuel and maintain a lean physique. This makes water fasting an effective tool for those looking to cleanse their bodies, lose weight, and improve their overall health.

Overall, the role of autophagy in anti-aging cannot be understated. By engaging in practices like water fasting, we can activate autophagy and promote cellular rejuvenation, ultimately leading to a longer, healthier, and more youthful life. So, for those looking to cleanse their bodies, lose weight, and slow down the aging process, incorporating water fasting and autophagy into their routine is a powerful and effective solution.

Reversing Aging Effects Through Autophagy

In the quest for eternal youth and vitality, many people are turning to the power of autophagy to reverse the aging effects on their bodies. Autophagy, which literally means "self-eating," is the body's natural process of breaking down and recycling damaged or dysfunctional cells and proteins. By stimulating autophagy through practices like water fasting, individuals can not only lose weight but also turn back the clock on aging.

Water fasting is a powerful tool for activating autophagy and promoting weight loss. By abstaining from food and only consuming water for a set period of time, the body is forced to rely on its stored fat for energy. This process not only helps shed excess pounds but also triggers autophagy, leading to the removal of toxins and damaged cells that contribute to aging.

For beginners looking to harness the benefits of autophagy and water fasting for weight loss, it is important to start slowly and gradually increase the duration of the fast. Starting with shorter fasts and gradually working up to longer periods can help the body adjust and maximize the effects of autophagy. Additionally, incorporating nutrient-dense foods before and after the fast can help support the body's natural detoxification processes.

One of the key benefits of autophagy is its anti-aging effects. By promoting cellular repair and regeneration, autophagy can help slow down the aging process and reduce the appearance of wrinkles, fine lines, and other signs of aging. By incorporating regular water fasting and autophagy practices into their routine, individuals can not only achieve their weight loss goals but also experience a more youthful and vibrant appearance.

In addition to its anti-aging benefits, autophagy has been shown to play a crucial role in disease prevention and overall health. By clearing out damaged cells and promoting healthy cell function, autophagy can help reduce the risk of chronic diseases such as cancer, diabetes, and heart disease. By embracing the power of autophagy through practices like water fasting, individuals can not only achieve their weight loss goals but also improve their overall health and well-being.

Chapter 6: Water Fasting for Mental Clarity and Focus

Enhancing Cognitive Function with Water Fasting

Water fasting has been known to have numerous benefits for the body, including enhancing cognitive function. When you abstain from food and only drink water, your body goes into a state of ketosis, where it begins to burn stored fat for energy. This process not only helps with weight loss but also has a positive impact on your brain function.

During water fasting, your body undergoes a process called autophagy, where it breaks down and recycles old or damaged cells. This process is particularly beneficial for the brain, as it helps to clear out toxins and improve overall cognitive function. Many people report feeling more focused and alert during a water fast, as their brain is able to function more efficiently without the burden of digesting food.

In addition to improving cognitive function, water fasting can also help to reset unhealthy eating habits. By taking a break from food and allowing your body to cleanse and detoxify, you can break the cycle of cravings and overeating. This can lead to long-term weight loss and improved overall health.

Furthermore, autophagy has been shown to have anti-aging benefits, as it helps to repair and rejuvenate cells throughout the body. By promoting this process through water fasting, you can not only look and feel younger but also protect against age-related cognitive decline.

Overall, incorporating water fasting into your weight loss and cleansing routine can have a profound impact on your cognitive function. By allowing your body to enter a state of ketosis and autophagy, you can improve mental clarity, focus, and overall brain health. So if you're looking to not only lose weight but also boost your brain power, consider adding water fasting to your wellness regimen.

Improving Mental Clarity Through Fasting

One of the lesser-known benefits of water fasting and autophagy is the significant improvement in mental clarity that many individuals experience during this process. Fasting allows the body to enter a state of ketosis, where it begins to burn fat for fuel instead of glucose. This shift in energy production can lead to increased mental clarity and focus, as the brain thrives on ketones produced during fasting.

For people that are trying to cleanse and lose weight, harnessing the power of mental clarity through fasting can be incredibly beneficial. When the mind is clear and focused, it becomes easier to make healthier food choices and resist cravings for unhealthy foods. This can lead to more successful weight loss and a greater sense of control over eating habits.

In addition to the cognitive benefits of fasting, autophagy plays a crucial role in supporting mental clarity. Autophagy is the body's natural process of cellular cleansing and recycling, which can help to remove damaged proteins and organelles from the brain. By promoting autophagy through fasting, individuals may experience improved cognitive function and protection against neurodegenerative diseases.

Furthermore, water fasting has been shown to reduce inflammation in the brain, which can contribute to improved mental clarity and focus. Chronic inflammation has been linked to cognitive decline and conditions such as Alzheimer's disease, so reducing inflammation through fasting may have long-term benefits for brain health.

Overall, incorporating water fasting and autophagy into a weight loss regimen can not only help individuals shed excess pounds but also improve mental clarity and focus. By allowing the body to enter a state of ketosis, promoting autophagy, and reducing inflammation in the brain, fasting can support cognitive function and enhance overall well-being. For those looking to cleanse, lose weight, and boost mental clarity, fasting may be a powerful tool to consider.

Chapter 7: Autophagy and Muscle Preservation During Fasting

Preserving Muscle Mass During Fasting

One of the biggest concerns for people embarking on a water fasting journey is the fear of losing muscle mass. While it is true that fasting can lead to muscle breakdown if not done correctly, there are ways to preserve muscle mass during fasting. By understanding the role of autophagy in the body, you can optimize your fasting experience to not only lose weight but also maintain your muscle mass.

Autophagy is a natural process in the body where damaged cells are broken down and recycled to create new, healthier cells. During fasting, autophagy is upregulated, which means that the body is more efficient at clearing out old and damaged cells. This process is crucial for preserving muscle mass during fasting, as it allows the body to break down and recycle damaged muscle cells while sparing healthy muscle tissue.

To preserve muscle mass during fasting, it is important to incorporate strength training exercises into your routine. By engaging in resistance training, you can stimulate muscle growth and prevent muscle breakdown during fasting. Additionally, consuming an adequate amount of protein before and after your fasting period can help support muscle repair and growth.

Another key factor in preserving muscle mass during fasting is to ensure you are getting enough rest and recovery. Sleep is essential for muscle repair and growth, so make sure to prioritize rest during your fasting journey. Additionally, staying hydrated and consuming electrolytes can help prevent muscle cramps and fatigue during fasting, allowing you to maintain your energy levels and continue exercising.

In conclusion, preserving muscle mass during fasting is possible with the right approach. By understanding the role of autophagy in the body and incorporating strength training exercises, adequate protein intake, and rest into your routine, you can optimize your fasting experience to not only lose weight but also maintain your muscle mass. Remember to listen to your body and make adjustments as needed to ensure a successful fasting journey.

Maintaining Strength Through Autophagy

Autophagy, the process by which your body cleanses itself of damaged cells and regenerates new ones, is a powerful tool in the fight against weight gain and disease. For people that are trying to cleanse and lose weight, harnessing the power of autophagy through water fasting can be a game changer. By allowing your body to enter a state of ketosis, where it burns fat for fuel instead of glucose, you can kickstart the autophagy process and begin to see real results in your weight loss journey.

One of the key benefits of autophagy during water fasting is its ability to preserve muscle mass. When you fast, your body naturally starts to break down muscle tissue for energy. However, by activating autophagy, you can target damaged or dysfunctional proteins within your muscle cells and recycle them for new growth. This not only helps you maintain your strength and stamina during fasting but also ensures that you are building lean muscle mass instead of losing it.

In addition to preserving muscle mass, autophagy has been shown to have anti-aging benefits that can help you look and feel younger. By clearing out old or damaged cells, autophagy promotes cellular rejuvenation and can help reduce the appearance of wrinkles, sagging skin, and other signs of aging. This is why many people who practice water fasting and autophagy report improvements in their skin tone, elasticity, and overall complexion.

Furthermore, autophagy plays a crucial role in disease prevention by helping to eliminate harmful toxins and free radicals from your body. When you fast, your body goes into a heightened state of autophagy, which allows it to target and remove damaged cells that could potentially lead to chronic illnesses such as cancer, diabetes, and heart disease. By incorporating regular water fasting and autophagy into your routine, you can significantly reduce your risk of developing these health conditions and enjoy a longer, healthier life.

Overall, maintaining strength through autophagy is essential for anyone looking to cleanse and lose weight. By understanding how autophagy works and how it can benefit your body, you can optimize your fasting regimen and achieve lasting results. Whether you are a beginner or an experienced faster, incorporating autophagy into your weight loss journey can help you reach your goals faster and more effectively than ever before.

Chapter 8: Water Fasting for Spiritual Growth

Connecting Mind, Body, and Spirit Through Water Fasting

In the quest for weight loss and overall well-being, many individuals are turning to water fasting as a means of cleansing their bodies and promoting autophagy. Water fasting involves abstaining from all food and consuming only water for a certain period of time, allowing the body to enter a state of deep detoxification and cellular repair. This process not only helps shed excess weight but also has a myriad of other health benefits that extend beyond physical appearance.

One of the key elements of water fasting is the connection it fosters between the mind, body, and spirit. By stripping away the distractions of food and focusing solely on hydration, individuals are able to tap into a deeper level of self-awareness and mindfulness. This heightened sense of presence can lead to a greater understanding of one's relationship with food and the emotional triggers that often accompany unhealthy eating habits.

Autophagy, the process by which the body cleans out damaged cells and regenerates new, healthy ones, is another key component of water fasting. This natural cellular repair mechanism is activated during periods of fasting, allowing the body to rid itself of toxins and waste that have accumulated over time. As a result, individuals may experience increased energy levels, improved mental clarity, and enhanced focus – all of which are essential for maintaining a healthy weight and lifestyle.

In addition to its physical benefits, water fasting has also been praised for its spiritual growth potential. Many individuals who embark on a fasting journey report feeling a sense of connection to something greater than themselves, whether it be through meditation, prayer, or simply quiet contemplation. This deepening of the spiritual self can provide a sense of purpose and clarity that extends far beyond the fasting period, helping individuals make positive changes in their lives long after the fast has ended.

Ultimately, connecting mind, body, and spirit through water fasting can be a transformative experience for those seeking to cleanse and lose weight. By embracing the power of autophagy and tapping into the deeper layers of consciousness that fasting provides, individuals can not only achieve their weight loss goals but also cultivate a greater sense of overall well-being and vitality. It is through this holistic approach to health and wellness that lasting change can be achieved, both physically and spiritually.

Enhancing Spiritual Awareness Through Fasting

Fasting has been utilized for centuries as a means of enhancing spiritual awareness and connecting with one's inner self. For individuals seeking to cleanse their bodies and shed excess weight, incorporating fasting into their routine can be a powerful tool. By abstaining from food and allowing the body to enter a state of autophagy, where it begins to break down and recycle damaged cells, individuals can experience a multitude of benefits beyond just weight loss.

One of the key ways in which fasting can enhance spiritual awareness is by promoting mindfulness and self-discipline. When we fast, we are forced to confront our desires and cravings, and learn to control them through willpower. This practice of self-control can help individuals develop a greater sense of inner strength and resilience, which can translate into other areas of their lives.

Fasting can also help individuals achieve a sense of mental clarity and focus, as the body is no longer preoccupied with digesting food. This heightened state of awareness can allow individuals to tap into their intuition and connect with their inner guidance, leading to a deeper sense of spiritual understanding and insight.

Furthermore, fasting can be a powerful tool for resetting unhealthy eating habits and breaking free from food addictions. By abstaining from food for a period of time, individuals can retrain their taste buds and reset their relationship with food, leading to healthier eating patterns and a greater sense of control over their diet.

Overall, incorporating fasting into a weight loss regimen can not only help individuals shed excess pounds, but also support their spiritual growth and enhance their overall well-being. By harnessing the power of autophagy and allowing the body to cleanse and rejuvenate itself, individuals can experience profound physical, mental, and spiritual benefits that can transform their lives for the better.

Chapter 9: Autophagy and Its Impact on Metabolism

Boosting Metabolism Through Autophagy

Boosting metabolism through autophagy is a powerful tool for those looking to cleanse and lose weight. Autophagy is the natural process by which the body breaks down and recycles old or damaged cells, leading to overall health improvements. By inducing autophagy through techniques such as water fasting, individuals can kickstart their metabolism and promote weight loss.

Water fasting is a popular method for initiating autophagy and boosting metabolism. By abstaining from food and consuming only water for a set period of time, the body is forced to rely on stored fat for energy, leading to weight loss. During a water fast, the body enters a state of ketosis, where it burns fat for fuel instead of carbohydrates. This process can increase metabolic rate and promote fat loss, making it an effective strategy for those looking to jumpstart their weight loss journey.

Autophagy plays a crucial role in weight loss by enhancing metabolism and promoting fat burning. When the body undergoes autophagy, it breaks down cellular components and recycles them for energy, leading to a more efficient metabolism. By inducing autophagy through techniques such as water fasting, individuals can optimize their metabolism and accelerate weight loss results. Additionally, autophagy can help preserve lean muscle mass during fasting, ensuring that weight loss comes primarily from fat stores.

In addition to its weight loss benefits, autophagy has been shown to have a range of other health benefits. By promoting cellular repair and regeneration, autophagy can help prevent age-related diseases and promote overall longevity. Water fasting, which induces autophagy, can also have anti-aging effects by promoting cellular rejuvenation and reducing oxidative stress. By incorporating autophagy into their weight loss journey through techniques such as water fasting, individuals can not only shed excess pounds but also improve their overall health and well-being.

Overall, boosting metabolism through autophagy is a powerful strategy for those looking to cleanse and lose weight. By inducing autophagy through techniques such as water fasting, individuals can kickstart their metabolism, promote fat burning, and accelerate weight loss results. In addition to its weight loss benefits, autophagy can also have a range of other health benefits, including anti-aging effects and disease prevention. By incorporating autophagy into their weight loss journey, individuals can optimize their metabolism, improve their overall health, and achieve their weight loss goals.

Improving Metabolic Health with Autophagy

For people that are trying to cleanse and lose weight, understanding the concept of autophagy and its impact on metabolic health can be a game-changer. Autophagy is a natural process in which the body cleans out damaged cells and regenerates new, healthy cells. This process is essential for maintaining optimal metabolic function and overall health.

One of the key benefits of autophagy for weight loss is its ability to regulate metabolism. By clearing out old, damaged cells, autophagy allows the body to function more efficiently, leading to increased energy levels and improved metabolism. This can help individuals reach their weight loss goals more quickly and effectively.

In addition to improving metabolism, autophagy can also play a role in preventing diseases associated with metabolic dysfunction, such as diabetes and heart disease. By promoting cellular regeneration and reducing inflammation, autophagy helps to protect against the development of these chronic conditions, making it an essential tool for maintaining long-term health.

When combined with water fasting, autophagy becomes even more powerful for improving metabolic health. Water fasting triggers autophagy by depriving the body of nutrients, forcing it to rely on its own resources for energy. This process not only enhances weight loss but also promotes cellular regeneration and detoxification, further supporting metabolic health.

Overall, incorporating autophagy into a weight loss regimen through practices like water fasting can lead to significant improvements in metabolic health. By promoting cellular regeneration, reducing inflammation, and enhancing metabolism, autophagy plays a crucial role in helping individuals cleanse their bodies, lose weight, and achieve optimal health.

Chapter 10: Water Fasting for Resetting Unhealthy Eating Habits

Breaking Bad Eating Habits Through Water Fasting

Breaking bad eating habits can be a challenging task, especially for those who have struggled with weight loss in the past. However, water fasting has been shown to be an effective method for breaking these habits and promoting weight loss. By abstaining from food and only consuming water for a set period of time, individuals can reset their unhealthy eating patterns and kickstart their journey towards a healthier lifestyle.

Water fasting is a powerful tool for detoxification, allowing the body to eliminate toxins and waste that have built up over time. This process can help to improve overall health and well-being, as well as promote weight loss. By giving the digestive system a break and allowing the body to focus on cleansing itself, water fasting can help individuals to break free from the cycle of unhealthy eating habits that may be holding them back from reaching their weight loss goals.

Autophagy, the process by which the body breaks down and recycles damaged cells, is another key benefit of water fasting. This natural cellular cleansing process is triggered during fasting and can help to promote weight loss by targeting stored fat for energy. By harnessing the power of autophagy through water fasting, individuals can not only lose weight but also improve their overall health and well-being.

In addition to weight loss, water fasting can also have a positive impact on mental clarity and focus. By giving the brain a break from the constant influx of food and allowing it to operate on ketones produced during fasting, individuals may experience increased concentration and cognitive function. This can be especially beneficial for those looking to break free from unhealthy eating habits and make better food choices in the future.

Overall, water fasting is a powerful tool for breaking bad eating habits and promoting weight loss. By harnessing the benefits of autophagy, detoxification, and improved mental clarity, individuals can reset their unhealthy patterns and pave the way for a healthier lifestyle. Whether you are looking to cleanse your body, lose weight, or improve your overall health, water fasting can be a transformative practice for achieving your goals.

Establishing Healthy Eating Patterns with Fasting

Fasting can be an incredibly powerful tool for cleansing the body and promoting weight loss, but it is essential to establish healthy eating patterns both during and after a fast to maximize the benefits. By incorporating fasting into your routine, you can reset unhealthy eating habits and kickstart your journey towards a healthier lifestyle.

One of the key benefits of fasting is its ability to promote autophagy, a natural process in which the body cleans out damaged cells and regenerates new, healthy ones. This can have a significant impact on weight loss, as it helps to boost metabolism and burn fat more efficiently. By establishing healthy eating patterns with fasting, you can enhance the autophagy process and accelerate your weight loss goals.

When embarking on a water fast for weight loss, it is important to focus on nutrient-dense foods during your eating windows. This means incorporating plenty of fruits, vegetables, whole grains, and lean proteins into your meals to ensure that your body is getting the essential nutrients it needs to support the fasting process. By fueling your body with healthy foods, you can optimize the effects of fasting and promote sustainable weight loss.

In addition to promoting weight loss, establishing healthy eating patterns with fasting can also have a positive impact on other aspects of your health, such as mental clarity, focus, and disease prevention. By nourishing your body with nutrient-dense foods, you can support brain function, improve concentration, and reduce your risk of chronic diseases. This makes fasting not only a powerful tool for weight loss, but also for overall health and wellness.

In conclusion, establishing healthy eating patterns with fasting is essential for anyone looking to cleanse their body, lose weight, and improve their overall health. By incorporating nutrient-dense foods into your meals, you can support the fasting process, promote autophagy, and achieve your weight loss goals more effectively. With a focus on healthy eating and fasting, you can reset unhealthy habits, boost your metabolism, and set yourself on the path towards a healthier, happier lifestyle.

Chapter 11: Autophagy and Its Role in Disease Prevention

Preventing Disease Through Autophagy

Autophagy is a natural process within our bodies that plays a crucial role in preventing disease and promoting overall health. By engaging in water fasting, you can effectively activate autophagy and harness its powerful benefits for weight loss and cleansing. Through the process of autophagy, damaged cells and toxins are broken down and recycled, leading to improved cellular function and reduced risk of chronic diseases such as cancer, diabetes, and heart disease.

Water fasting is a powerful tool for kickstarting the autophagy process in your body. By abstaining from food for a set period of time, you can stimulate autophagy and promote the elimination of harmful substances that may be lurking in your cells. This can lead to weight loss, improved detoxification, and increased energy levels. By incorporating regular water fasting into your routine, you can support your body in its natural ability to prevent disease and maintain optimal health.

For those new to water fasting, it is important to start slowly and gradually increase the duration of your fasts as your body becomes accustomed to the process. By allowing your body to adapt to the fasting state, you can maximize the benefits of autophagy and achieve your weight loss goals more effectively. Remember to stay hydrated during your fasts and listen to your body's signals to ensure a safe and successful experience.

In addition to its role in weight loss and cleansing, autophagy has been shown to have a profound impact on aging and disease prevention. By activating autophagy through water fasting, you can support your body in its ability to repair and regenerate cells, leading to improved longevity and reduced risk of age-related illnesses. Incorporating regular water fasting into your routine can help you harness the anti-aging benefits of autophagy and maintain a youthful and vibrant appearance.

Overall, by embracing the power of autophagy through water fasting, you can take control of your health and well-being. By preventing disease, promoting weight loss, and supporting cellular regeneration, you can achieve your goals for cleansing and rejuvenation. With dedication and consistency, you can unlock the transformative benefits of autophagy and experience a renewed sense of vitality and vitality.

Strengthening the Immune System with Autophagy

Autophagy is a natural process in the body that helps to cleanse and repair damaged cells, ultimately strengthening the immune system. When we engage in practices like water fasting, we are able to trigger autophagy more effectively, leading to numerous health benefits. For people that are trying to cleanse and lose weight, understanding how autophagy works can be a game changer in achieving their goals.

During a water fast, the body is deprived of food, forcing it to rely on stored energy sources. This process not only helps with weight loss, but it also activates autophagy, allowing the body to break down and recycle old and damaged cells. By strengthening the immune system through autophagy, individuals can experience improved overall health and vitality.

Autophagy plays a crucial role in detoxification, as it helps to eliminate toxins and waste products from the body. By promoting the removal of harmful substances, autophagy can support the liver and other detoxification pathways, leading to a more efficient cleansing process. This is particularly important for individuals looking to reset unhealthy eating habits and jumpstart their weight loss journey.

In addition to its detoxification benefits, autophagy has also been shown to have anti-aging effects. By removing damaged cells and promoting the regeneration of healthy ones, autophagy can help to slow down the aging process and improve skin health. This is why many people turn to water fasting and other autophagy-inducing practices as a way to maintain a youthful appearance and feel more energized.

Overall, understanding how autophagy works and incorporating practices like water fasting into your routine can have a profound impact on your health and well-being. By strengthening the immune system through autophagy, individuals can support weight loss, detoxification, anti-aging benefits, and more. For those looking to cleanse, lose weight, and improve their overall health, harnessing the power of autophagy is a powerful tool that can lead to lasting results.

Chapter 12: Conclusion

Recap of Water Fasting and Autophagy Benefits

In this subchapter, we will recap the incredible benefits of water fasting and autophagy for those who are seeking to cleanse their bodies and lose weight. Water fasting is a powerful tool for detoxification, weight loss, mental clarity, and spiritual growth. By abstaining from food and consuming only water for a set period of time, the body is able to tap into its natural healing mechanisms and rid itself of toxins and excess fat.

Autophagy, which is the body's natural process of cellular renewal, is also heavily stimulated during water fasting. This process allows the body to break down and recycle old and damaged cells, leading to improved overall health and anti-aging benefits. Autophagy is also crucial for preserving muscle mass during fasting, as the body prioritizes the breakdown of dysfunctional cells over healthy muscle tissue.

One of the key benefits of water fasting and autophagy is their impact on metabolism. By giving the digestive system a break and allowing the body to burn stored fat for energy, fasting can help reset the metabolism and promote weight loss. Additionally, autophagy has been shown to play a role in disease prevention, as it helps the body eliminate harmful cells that can lead to chronic illnesses.

For beginners looking to try water fasting, it is important to start slowly and gradually increase the fasting period over time. It is also essential to stay hydrated and listen to your body's signals throughout the process. Fasting can be a challenging experience, both physically and mentally, but the benefits are well worth the effort. By incorporating water fasting and autophagy into your routine, you can achieve not only weight loss but also improved overall health and well-being.

Final Thoughts on Using Fasting for Cleansing and Weight Loss

In conclusion, incorporating fasting into your routine can be a powerful tool for both cleansing and weight loss. Whether you choose to do a water fast or practice autophagy through intermittent fasting, the benefits are clear. By allowing your body to enter a state of ketosis, you can kickstart your metabolism and burn fat more efficiently. Additionally, the process of autophagy can help to detoxify your cells and promote overall health.

It is important to remember that fasting is not a one-size-fits-all solution. It is crucial to listen to your body and consult with a healthcare professional before embarking on any fasting regimen. Fasting can be challenging, especially for beginners, so it is important to start slowly and gradually build up your fasting times. Remember to stay hydrated and nourish your body with nutrient-dense foods during non-fasting periods to support your overall health and well-being.

Furthermore, fasting is not just about physical benefits, but can also have positive effects on your mental and spiritual well-being. Many people report increased mental clarity and focus during fasting, as well as a sense of spiritual growth and connection. By taking the time to reset your eating habits and give your digestive system a break, you can cultivate a deeper awareness of your body and its needs.

In addition to weight loss and cleansing, fasting can also play a role in disease prevention and anti-aging. The process of autophagy helps to remove damaged cells and promote cellular repair, which can reduce the risk of chronic diseases and slow down the aging process. By incorporating fasting into your lifestyle, you can support your body in maintaining optimal health and vitality.

Overall, fasting can be a powerful tool for anyone looking to cleanse their body, lose weight, and improve their overall health. By understanding the principles of water fasting and autophagy, you can harness the benefits of these practices to support your wellness goals. Remember to approach fasting with mindfulness, patience, and self-care, and you may be amazed at the transformative results it can bring to your life.

www.ingramcontent.com/pod-product-compliance
Lightning Source LLC
Chambersburg PA
CBHW081545250726
48659CB00009B/3088